DOG TRAINING FOR AGGRESSIVE DOGS

AGGRESSIVE DOG TRAINING GUIDE FOR BEGINNERS

DINA KELLY

COPYRIGHT

Copyright © 2021 by DINA KELLY: All rights reserved. This book or any portion thereof may not be reproduced or used in any manner whatsoever without the express written permission of the author except for the use of brief quotations in a book review.

TABLE OF CONTENTS

INTRODUCTION 5

CHAPTER ONE 7

Major Causes of Aggression in Dogs 7

CHAPTER TWO 11

How to Reduce Consistent Barking in Dogs 11

CHAPTER THREE 14

Basic Home Training for Dogs 14

CHAPTER FOUR 17

How to Train Your Dog to Stay 17

CHAPTER FIVE 19

How to treat minor separation anxiety 19

CHAPTER SIX 22

Aggressive Triggeers in Dogs 22

CHAPTER SEVEN 25

DOG TRAINING TREATS 25

CHAPTER EIGHT 29

POSITIVE REINFORCEMENT IN DOG TRAINING 29

CHAPTER NINE 31

CALMING TREATS 31

CHAPTER TEN 33

PUPPY TRAINING: HOME OR AWAY 33
TAKING REST PERIODS 35

CONCLUSION 37

INTRODUCTION

Aggression is difficult to fix without the root cause, part of the difficulty stems from the fact that there are several different types of dog aggression, such as predatory, dominant, territorial, food, sexual, fear, and so on, as well as the fact that some normal socialization behaviours, such as barking, biting, growling, jumping, and so on, can appear aggressive. Aggression can be considerably reduced or eliminated with regular interaction and training. Detecting symptoms of aggressiveness, on the other hand, is critical. The most evident and potentially harmful aspects of aggression are dominance, assertiveness, and fear.

Aggression is a challenging condition to diagnose! This book would assist you in keeping your dog quiet and healthy. I strongly advise anyone who owns a dog that displays signs of aggression, or even if they are unsure, to get professional help.

Predatory aggression, sexual aggression, and territorial aggression are examples of aggressive dog behaviours that should not be overlooked and must be addressed. Furthermore, food or toy antagonism can be extremely dangerous, particularly for youngsters, and must be addressed. This book will help you better understand your dog so that your home is free of hostility.

CHAPTER ONE

Major Causes of Aggression in Dogs

Anxiety in dogs is a natural fear response gone awry. The fight, flight, freeze response is a healthy and important survival skill when it is triggered in response to a real threat, but anxiety occurs when it is triggered in anticipation of something that cannot harm you such as; thunder, fireworks, sudden loud noises, a new environment, or even visual stimuli like hats and umbrellas. Anxiety in pets can be caused by a variety of factors, including puppy socialization challenges, age-related health concerns such as dementia, traumatic experiences, or heredity. Separation anxiety, one of the most common causes of stress in dogs, is another source of anxiety in dogs. Separation anxiety has been connected to dogs that have spent time in shelters, been roaming the streets, or have a history of abandonment; it can be caused by a change in routine, family members joining or departing the household, and/or simply being left alone for any length of time.

Fear: Aggressive behaviour can quickly develop in a terrified dog. Most dogs only become aggressive when they perceive themselves to be in danger, are unable to flee, and feel compelled to defend themselves. This could happen if a dog is in a scary situation, for instance, in a corner with no way out, or if he believes a handheld over his head implies he'll be hit. If your dog is a rescue dog who is more aggressive or scared than usual, it may have been abused, neglected, had a traumatic occurrence, or was not properly socialized as a puppy. Any information you can obtain from the organization where you acquired the dog could assist you in determining the best course of action. Rescue dogs may require obedience training from a trainer who specializes in educating dogs who have been abused or who have not been properly socialized. With training and patience, you may be able to handle your dog's fear on your own in some circumstances. A veterinarian can advise you on the best course of action. Approach unknown dogs with caution to prevent encouraging aggressive behaviour, let them approach you without feeling scared of the unknown. To assist your dog to avoid fear in the future, train and socialize him.

Pain: Dogs have emotions. Pain is a very common source of hostility for dogs. Your suddenly aggressive dog could be suffering from an injury or disease that is giving him a lot of pain and worry. Arthritis, bone fractures, internal traumas, tumors, and lacerations are all possible causes of pain.

Possessiveness: When a dog is possessive of something, possession aggression, also known as resource guarding, arises. Possessive aggression can be noticed in these areas: food, toys, or some other valuable item. When someone approaches his food bowl or gets too close while he is chewing a favourite toy, a dog with possession aggression may growl. A dog may also bite a stranger who enters the dog's territory, which is your home. Aggression levels differ from one dog to the next and between items. For example, your dog may not mind if you sit down and pet him as he chews a rubber toy, but if you do the same thing while he chews a pig's ear, he may turn and snap at you. It all depends on how much each object or resource is valued by the dog.

Illness: Ailments can influence your dog's brain, causing him to act irrationally aggressively. Aggression can be triggered by conditions such as cognitive impairment, brain disorders, or malignancies. These issues are more common in older dogs, but they can develop at any age. Before attempting to treat your dog's sudden, unexplained aggression as a behaviour problem, consult your veterinarian. You might be tempted to give your dog pain medicine, but this is something you should avoid. If your dog is sick, you'll need to figure out exactly what's wrong before you start treating it. Don't try to handle things on your own until you've figured out what you're up against. Only a veterinarian can advise you on the best drugs for your dog.

CHAPTER TWO

How to Reduce Consistent Barking in Dogs

When your dog continues to bark for no apparent reason, you must determine the source of the problem and address it as soon as possible. Dogs are a person's best friend however, they can become aggressive due to unanticipated circumstances. Let's look into some options for reducing our dogs' constant barking.

Simple Is Best: Dogs can be taught to understand particular words, but it's crucial to stick to your directions. Choose your favourite synonym for "quiet," but make sure you use the same word every time you want your dog to stay quiet.

Don't Retaliate Against Your Dog: You might be inclined to raise your voice when you're frustrated. But always resist the desire; your dog may believe you're partaking in the barking, which may make him bark even louder. Instead, use a quiet, soothing tone of speech.

Identify the Barking Problem's Root Cause: Dogs bark for a variety of reasons, and some are particularly vocal when defending what they perceive to be their territory. When a person or another animal comes too close, your pet may feel obligated to tell them they're not welcome. Barking can also be a sign of loneliness, separation anxiety, or fear in dogs.

Reduce Dog Barking by Limiting Stimuli Exposure: Limiting exposure to external stimuli for territorial barkers can be as simple as closing window curtains while you're away or building a privacy fence for outside dogs. Dogs have been hearing, so the sounds of people or animals approaching on their territory may still stimulate them, but limiting their capacity to watch the action may be beneficial.

Recognize and reward good behaviour: Dogs have no idea that their barking irritates you or causes your neighbours to file noise complaints with the police department. Treats, on the other hand, are a no-brainer for your dog. Use your one-word order calmly when your dog is barking. Reward him with a goodie as soon as he comes to a halt.

Stopping Dog Barking Requires Exercise: There is are scientific evidence that exercise is one of the most effective ways to relieve stress, and it's also a wonderful treatment for worried animals. Ensure that your dog gets enough exercise each day. If at all feasible, schedule the training session to coincide with the usual issue barking periods. You can also get in a good stroll or a trip to the park before work, which is a lovely way to start the day.

Give Your Dog a Physical Exam: Although barking is a typical part of a dog's temperament, excessive vocalization could suggest a medical problem. It's a good idea to take your previously quiet pet to your veterinarian for a check-up if he or she has suddenly started making a lot of noise.

Put a stop to the barking: Allowing your dog to bark for an extended period can reinforce the behaviour. It is always better to deal with barking problems as soon as they emerge rather than allowing your pet to become accustomed to it.

CHAPTER THREE

Basic Home Training for Dogs

One of the strategies to develop regular positive habits is to train at home. We may give our dogs or other pets home instruction in the same way we train our children to help them develop good habits. The following are some helpful hints for teaching your dog some basic commands.

Excitement: If your dog is still having accidents in the house, it could be something more serious than a simple housebreaking problem. Teach your dog to feel at home and do things right around the home.

Dogs and Puppies on the Leash: Every dog should be taught to walk on a leash. Apart from the fact that leash restrictions exist in most locations, there will be situations when keeping your dog on a leash is necessary for his protection. Learn how to introduce your dog or puppy to the leash, then show him how to walk on it properly, even while riding a bike behind you. Walking on a loose leash teaches your dog not to pull or lunge when on the leash, making the experience more enjoyable for both you and your dog.

Dogs and Puppies Crate Training: Here are the fundamentals of teaching your dog or puppy to tolerate and even like their crate. It will not only assist with home keeping but will also provide your dog with his own space. When it comes down to it, house training your dog isn't all that difficult, but that doesn't mean it's simple. During the housebreaking process, consistency and diligence are essential.

Home training for your dog: Unless you intend to keep your dog outside which few of us do because it's not recommended. You would need to teach your dog where to go potty. As a result, one of the first things you should work on with your dog is home training, potty training is one of the essential areas. Home training can be a highly beneficial component of your dog's training. This involves both house training and a variety of different types of training listed below.

How to Socialize Puppies and Dogs: By exposing your puppy or adult dog to different people, animals, and environments, you may teach him to tolerate new people, creatures, and places. Dogs who have been socialized are less prone to develop behavioural issues and are generally more well-liked by their peers. Socialization can also aid in the prevention of phobias and fears. In the end, socializing with your dog or puppy will make him a happier and better-behaved pup.

Basic Instructions and Tricks: Every dog should know some basic dog training commands and skills, such as come, speak, drop it, stay, back up, and so on. Basic commands provide structure for your dog. They can also assist you in overcoming common dog behaviour issues and keeping your dog safe.

Using a Clicker to Train Dogs: Clicker training is a simple and successful dog training approach that uses positive reinforcement. Although you may train your dog without using a clicker, many people find it beneficial. You can easily and efficiently teach your dog all types of basic and advanced instructions and tricks with clicker training. Learning how to clicker train your dog is simple and quick.

CHAPTER FOUR

How to Train Your Dog to Stay

Nothing beats showing off your dog's impressive abilities. Dog tricks are a fantastic method to take your dog's training to the next level while also providing mental stimulation for your dog. Proofing is a further step in teaching your dog a new trick. Learn how to proof behaviours so that your dog is as obedient at the park or at a friend's house as he is at home. Remember that just because you've gone through several dog training doesn't mean you won't run across behavioural issues. Put your skills to the test in a variety of circumstances with varying degrees of distraction. If you don't proof your dog, he may behave beautifully in your living room but seem to forget everything he's learned when he's outside. Discover the most frequent dog behaviour issues and how to handle them. These guides will assist you in navigating this stage of the training with your dog.

Teach Your Dog Self-Control: This strategy teaches your dog that nothing in life comes for free, and that food and attention must be earned via obedience.

Dog Behaviour Management vs. Dog Training: While these two concepts are distinct, they are not mutually exclusive. Any dog training program should include behaviour control.

Common Dog Behaviour Issues: Recognizing and addressing potential behavioural issues might help you catch them before they spiral out of hand.

CHAPTER FIVE

How to treat minor separation anxiety

When dogs with separation anxiety are left alone, they experience suffering and behavioural issues. Some of the more common methods include: Attempting to reconcile with their owners by digging and scratching at doors or windows, chewing that causes damage, whining, howling and barking, defecation and urination. It's unclear why some dogs experience separation anxiety while others do not. However, keep in mind that your dog's actions are part of a panic response. Your dog isn't attempting to reprimand you! They simply want you to return home! Some examples of situations that can cause separation anxiety: For the first time being left alone, being alone when you're used to having a continual human touch. Being subjected to a traumatic incident, such as being confined to a shelter or boarding kennel, loss of a family member or other pet, or a change in the family's routine or structure. Arrivals and departures should not be celebrated; instead, ignore your dog for the first several minutes before softly petting them. Leave your dog with recently worn clothes that have a strong resemblance to yours. Establish a statement or action that informs your dog you'll be returning every time you leave. Consider using an over-the-counter relaxing product to help your dog become less anxious. Here are some suggestions for dealing with minimal separation anxiety.

Safe Place: Use the above strategies in conjunction with desensitization training. Use positive reinforcement to teach your dog the sit-stay and down-stay commands. This training will teach them how to remain calm and happy in one location as they move to another. To minimize your dog's potential to be destructive while you're away, create a "safe place." A secure location should include the following features: Keep the dog in loose confinement; a room with a window and toys, not total isolation, Provide distractions in the form of busy toys, have filthy clothing or other safety cues to provide a relaxing fragrance.

How to deal with your dog when he or she is learning to be calm: Your dog's terror response to your departures may take some time to unlearn. Consider the following interim remedies to assist you and your dog cope in the short term: Consult your veterinarian about medication therapy to help them cope with their anxiousness, if you have to go away, leave your dog in doggie daycare or kennel, when you're gone, leave your dog with a friend, family member, or neighbour, if at all feasible, bring your dog to work with you.

CHAPTER SIX
AGGRESSIVE TRIGGEERS IN DOGS

It's difficult to understand why your dog has suddenly turned nasty, especially if he was previously kind. His rage could be aimed at his owner, odd individuals, or other animals. Given the numerous causes of canine aggression, you must first determine the source of the problem before developing a solution.

Triggers of Fear: Fear is simple to comprehend. It has the ability to bring out the worst in both people and animals. When your dog feels threatened, he will use every weapon at his disposal to defend himself, including barking and biting. It's important to remember that this is about your dog's perceptions, not necessarily reality. Even if it has nothing to do with your pet, a sudden gesture can be interpreted as unfriendly. Attempting to steal something the dog values, reaching or bending over his body, maintaining eye contact, or attempting to physically relocate him are all common triggers of fear aggression.

Competition: Dogs who reside in the same house are often seen as pack members, but it does not imply they will not fight. Canines in the wild establish supremacy by fighting one another. Domesticated dogs have the same instinct as wild dogs. Once the order is established, the hostility should subside, but your dog will always be vigilant of challenges to his authority. Dominance-related aggression can be triggered by holding your dog, occupying one of his favourite locations, interrupting his sleep, or interfering with him while he feeds. Separate your dog from all other people and animals when you feed him if he is particularly violent at mealtimes.

Territorial Conflict: Boundaries are important to dogs. They will battle to defend their space and will not allow intrusions. It's in their nature, and it's very impossible to entirely condition them out of it. While not all dogs attack strangers or other animals, you should always be prepared for them to do so. When your dog goes outside, keep him confined behind a towering fence or on a safe leash. You could be a victim of territorial aggression. If your dog believes that another person is attempting to harm you or your family, he may attack them. If a stranger speaks to you in a loud or angry tone or makes a potentially threatening move, your pet may bite to protect his "pack."

Additional Triggers: Dogs, like people, are unique individuals. They remember what occurred to them and may have psychological issues as a result. They may react violently when exposed to the stimuli again if they have been abused or damaged by anything or someone in their lives. It's impossible to forecast these triggers, but if you find that a certain stimulation irritates your pet, don't expose him to it again. Your pet may become aggressive as a result of redirected aggression. When your dog can't get to the cause of his rage, such as a dog he sees through a window, or when someone intervenes in a fight between him and another dog, this form of violence occurs.

CHAPTER SEVEN
Dog Training Treats

There are numerous methods for rewarding your dog for a job well done. Throwing a tennis ball at the conclusion of a long "stay" or a romp in the backyard after practising "wait" by the door might be a good idea. However, the easiest and successful way to influence your dog's behaviour is through food treats. Here are some pointers on selecting the best dog treat for the situation.

Fast-Food Snacks: It's critical to keep your dog engaged and interested when teaching him new actions. A high rate of reinforcement is one of the simplest methods to accomplish this (how often you give rewards). You'll need to find goodies that your dog can eat rapidly if you want to give him a lot of rewards in a short amount of time. If your dog eats his treat right away, you can move on to the following repetition. He maintains his attention and gains a great deal of practice in a short period of time. However, if your dog takes several seconds to consume each reward, you'll have to wait longer between repetitions. You'll have to either lengthen your training sessions and risk losing your dog's attention or perform fewer repetitions every session.

Treats that are both soft and stinky: Soft dog treats are also useful for training because they are easier and faster for your dog to eat than crunchy ones. Biscuits are wonderful for one-time rewards, but waiting for your dog to discover every crumbled piece on the floor during a training session takes time away from teaching. Never forget to give your pet soft snacks. Every dog has a reward hierarchy, and most of them would prioritize stinky foods like cheese or bacon. In your calm living room, you might be able to get away with using kibble as a reward, but in a more distracting area, you should use the stinky treats your dog loves.

Treats should be kept small: Small dog treats are essential for moving a training session forward. Even huge dogs will be satisfied with a pea-sized treat. You can use even smaller pieces for little dogs. Some store-bought snacks are far too big. Before you begin your training session, look for tiny treats or cut larger ones into small pieces. You may feel like you're cheating your dog, but as long as he gets something he likes, he won't mind whether it's a nibble or the entire wiener. Smaller snacks are also easier for your dog's stomach. Your dog may be eating handfuls of treats every day, especially when training is rigorous, such as with pups or dogs preparing for certain sports. Smaller goodies imply fewer calories are consumed. It also ensures that your puppy will not become overly full before the lesson ends.

Adding Variety: Your dog may like a range of treats, just as he may prefer some treats over others. With the same old treat, dogs can become bored. If your dog's excitement wanes, switch to a different incentive of equal or greater value. You can also use a variety of rewards during a training session, so your dog never knows what kind of tasty morsel to expect next.

Slow-Cooking Recipes: Treats should sometimes be kept as long as feasible. Teaching your dog to enjoy his kennel, keeping him occupied while you're gone, or encouraging him to lie calmly alongside you as you watch TV are all ideal scenarios for a long-lasting reward. Look for chewy goodies that your dog will enjoy, such as bully sticks. Use dog toys that can be stuffed with food as an alternative. For a time-consuming treat, a Kong might be stuffed with cream cheese or peanut butter. Alternatively, plug the end, fill it with broth, and freeze it for a refreshing snack on a hot day.

Food in Your Pocket: Treats are useful for spontaneous training, such as praising positive behaviour around the house, such as lying quietly on a dog bed. Having food in your pocket or a dog treat bag with you at all times will allow you to deliver an immediate incentive in these situations. Perishable delicacies, such as leftover chicken, will not suffice. Look for goodies that are non-perishable and easy to transport, such as freeze-dried liver or jerky treats sliced into small pieces.

CHAPTER EIGHT

Positive Reinforcement in Dog Training

In order to get the desired results, dog training necessitates patience and persistence. Positive reinforcement may aid in the development of consistent positive habits in your dog and the transition from aggression to good conduct. Positive reinforcement is an excellent method for teaching your dog commands and reinforcing positive behaviour. You can have your dog sit for you if you want: Before allowing them to go out, this would prevent door slamming, before you pet them, before you feed them, this could help teach good mealtime manners. Give them a pat or a "good dog" if they lie peacefully at your feet, or give them a reward toy to chew on instead of your shoe. I would talk about the greatest techniques to help your dog understand and communicate with you better in this chapter.

It's all about the timing: When applying positive reinforcement, it's critical to get the timing right. If the incentive isn't given right away within seconds, your pet may not associate it with the right behaviour. If you ask your dog to sit but then treat them when they stand back up, they will believe they are being rewarded for standing.

Keep it brief: Dogs are unable to comprehend language. "Dainty, I'd like you to be a good girl and sit for me right now," you'll probably get a blank stare. In reality, dogs pick up on our body language first, so practice coaxing your dog into a "sit" or "down" before approaching them with a command. Start adding the word "sit" or "down" if they've worked out the behaviour regularly, but don't repeat it and say it in a calm manner. Keep orders simple and straightforward. The following are the most regularly used dog commands: sit, stay, stand, come, leave, stop, go buddy and several others.

Consistency is essential: Otherwise, your dog may become confused if everyone in the family uses the same commands. It could be beneficial to post a list of commands so that everyone is familiar with them. Consistency also implies that the desired behaviour is always rewarded and the undesirable behaviour is never rewarded.

CHAPTER NINE

Calming Treats

Calming treats which contain herbs and vitamins as active components, are a non-medicinal anxiety-relieving cure you can give your dog to help alleviate her symptoms. Nutraceuticals, often known as calming chews or calming bites, are nutritional supplements for people that are similar to calming chews or bites. Dogs are carnivores by nature, and while there is no evidence that these herbs are dangerous to pets, relaxing treats containing them often lack proof that animals will react to them in the same manner that humans do. Other botanical elements in soothing treats, such as lavender or ginger, have long been known to be relaxing for people but haven't been thoroughly researched for usage in animals. Tryptophan and melatonin, two active substances typically present in soothing foods, have been shown to have more verified relaxing effects. Other ingredients include the amino acid L-Theanine which is thought to work by increasing your dog's serotonin and dopamine levels, as well as probiotics, which are thought to support digestive health as well as a positive mental state and help with dogs who get diarrhoea when stressed.

Treats are an important part of a happy and healthy dog's life. Use a variety of healthy snacks to train your puppy. Many puppy owners are overwhelmed in the first few weeks after bringing their new pet home. There are supplies to be purchased, appointments to be made, and a great deal of training to be completed. It's crucial to establish the correct behaviours and expectations early on in your puppy's life, and puppy obedience training programs are a great place to start. Choosing the best obedience training lessons for you and your dog depends on a number of things. Distance is undoubtedly important; but, convenience should not be the only factor influencing your decision. Other factors to consider include training methods, relevant lessons for your needs, compatibility of the instructor's personality with yours, and the instructor's certificates.

CHAPTER TEN

Puppy Training: Home or Away

There are advantages to both home and group training. Some personal trainers will come to your home and provide one-on-one instruction. Some dog owners choose to train their puppy themselves. You and your dog may be able to focus more on each other if you train at home. Even though there are distractions from other dogs, group class training helps your dog learn to focus. One advantage of home training is that it is private; you and your trainer can concentrate on the skills you want your dog to master, whereas group classes may spend time on topics you don't care about. You may have no alternative but to train at home in some situations; distant or rural areas may lack a local training institution where you can enroll in group lessons.

Arousal: Pets have emotions. Arousal is a fantastic place to start. We enable our dog's hyperactive behaviour without even realizing it. Our dogs, for example, bark out the windows, fight over the fence, and visit dog parks. The chemicals released during arousal can last up to twenty-four hours in our dog's system. Then we wonder why our dogs are so agitated. Here are a few suggestions. If your dog barks at everything that moves outside the home, use baby gates to keep him out of the room with the large picture window, close the blinds, or install Decorative Arts window film that allows you to look out but not your dog. You can use classical music or a white noise machine to block out part of the disturbance if you know when your dog is stimulated for example, when the bus drops off kids after school or the trash trucks make their rounds. Instead of going to the dog park, play fetch or tug with one compatible buddy or arrange a playdate.

Choosing an Instructor for Obedience Training: Most training institutes will gladly allow you to observe a class or two to ensure that the teaching approach is compatible with your views, leave your pup at home for this. Most dogs learn best through positive reinforcement training, which involves praising the dog for making the proper decision while withholding rewards or ignoring the dog when the dog makes the wrong option.

Default Actions: Your dog's default behaviours are what he does when he doesn't know what else to do. Have pea-sized snacks in your pocket or treat bag or stowed throughout the house to teach a default behaviour, such as sit or down. When you see your dog doing something you like, the rewards come out. Keep in mind that you are not commanding your dog to sit. You're rewarding your dog for something he does on his own. Because he has been praised for sitting, your dog will begin to sit more frequently. After that, the treats can become more random, and if it's evident that sit is your dog's usual habit, you can start substituting a belly rub or a toy for the food reward. What is it about sitting as a default action that is so appealing? Consider this: how often have you seen a dog sitting "over the top"? Sitting is the first step toward relaxation, and it's what we call an "incompatible" activity.

Assisting your dog to unwind after a training session: How many of you with high-energy dogs wish you could spend time cooking supper, talking on the phone, or reading the mail without ripping up cushions to attract your attention. Although some dogs have higher levels of activity than others (think teenage dogs), it is beneficial for all dogs to learn to settle down. You might be surprised to learn that soothing behaviour can be learned. Indeed, there are so many different strategies to teach soothing behaviour that it can be difficult to know where to begin.

Taking Rest Periods: Yes, dogs require exercise, and we don't mean a leisurely stroll. Too much stimulation without a pause, on the other hand, is a recipe for disaster. If your dog can run in your yard with a pal, play fetch (even down the stairs), chase bubbles, pull or get through your homemade obstacle course, that's fantastic. But don't forget to take frequent breaks and stop having fun. This not only reduces your dog's arousal level, but also teaches him to shift from enthusiasm to calm. Allow your dog to play some more after a break so that he would be more willing to take following breaks without complaining. If your dog is too preoccupied to listen, you don't want to call him away from his playtime. Your dog will be more likely to come to you in a peaceful place after you have a 100 percent dependable recall inside, especially if he has learned from experience that coming to you doesn't always signal the end of fun. Go get him until then.

CONCLUSION

Your dog won't be able to tell you when or why he or she is worried, but her behaviour will give you signs. Here are a few hints: Aggression, urinating or defecating in a public place, drooling, panting, negative behaviour, depression, an excessive amount of barking, pacing, restlessness, compulsive or repetitive habits

There are times when you may be able to quickly identify and cure the source of your dog's anxiety e.g., situation avoidance, regular exercise and stimulation, or behavioural or obedience training, but on other occasions, your dog's anxiety may be completely beyond your control. You might wish to look for an alternative solution in certain situations.

www.ingramcontent.com/pod-product-compliance
Lightning Source LLC
Chambersburg PA
CBHW070904220526
45466CB00005B/2128